VITAMIN D, VITAMIN C AND IODINE

WHAT TO BE AWARE OF

BILLIE J. GREEN

DISCLAIMER

Copyright © 2023 Billie J. Green.

TABLE OF CONTENTS

INTRODUCTION

Iodine, vitamin C, and vitamin D are three extraordinarily amazing nutrients that support wellness. This book explains how these three can be used to prevent, treat, and even cure several illnesses and medical disorders.

It explains how to use these substances safely while avoiding using them excessively.

Who is this book intended for? Anyone who desires to lead a life free from diseases and health issues.

CHAPTER ONE

VITAMIN D

In addition to being necessary for strong bones, vitamin D (also known as calciferol) may also support the immune system and other bodily processes. Vitamin D is produced in the human body as a reaction to sun exposure. A person can raise their vitamin D intake by eating certain foods or taking supplements.

For strong bones and teeth, vitamin D is essential. In addition, it performs a variety of other important functions in the body, such as domineering immune reaction and inflammation.

Regardless of its name, vitamin D is a hormone or prohormone and not a vitamin.

A National Health and Nutrition Examination Survey found that 61% of children under the age of 21 and 40% of adults in the United States have low vitamin D levels. According to other sources, one billion people worldwide and three out of four Americans are believed to be vitamin D deficient.

Women, Black Americans, and anyone with a higher body mass index are at a higher risk of having low vitamin D levels. Living in areas where natural sunlight may be scarce (especially in winter), air pollution, and not eating enough vitamin D-rich foods like salmon, tuna, fortified orange juice, egg yolk, cheese, mushroom, and mutton are all thought to contribute to inadequate vitamin D levels. Vitamin D is a nutrient crucial for immune function, bone and heart health, disease prevention, and more. Many bodily processes as well as the treatment and prevention of numerous diseases depend on vitamin D.

CANCER

The Garland brothers conducted the first study in the 1990s, relating latitude and colon cancer risk, and then they conducted a prospective study on vitamin D status and colon cancer risk.

They came to two conclusions. The first is that your risk of developing colorectal cancer increases with latitude. They also concluded that daily vitamin D intake of 1,000 units may lower colon cancer risk by as much as 50%. In accordance with various studies, increasing your vitamin D status has the potential to reduce the risk of colorectal cancer by 25% to 50%.

The National Cancer Institute also states in a report that "numerous epidemiological studies have shown that higher intake or blood levels of vitamin D are associated with a reduced risk of colorectal cancer." Dr. Knight conducted an excellent study in Canada. She conducted a telephone survey of Canadian women who had breast cancer and a similar survey of Canadian women in the same region who had no such disease. She concluded that women who spent the most time in the sun as teenagers and young adults had a nearly 70% lower risk of developing breast cancer later in life. Therefore, there is sufficient evidence to conclude that increasing vitamin D status can lower the risk of breast cancer.

INFECTION

Numerous epidemiological studies in both adults and children have shown that vitamin D deficiency increases the risk and severity of infection, especially respiratory infections.

According to recent research, vitamin D significantly affects gene expression that affects the immune system and the inflammatory cascade.

Through a variety of mechanisms, vitamin D seems to affect both the likelihood of infection and its severity.

It affects cytokine profiles during infection via the innate and adaptive immune systems, and it directly affects the production of the antimicrobial peptide cathelicidin, which may increase susceptibility to viruses and bacteria.

Consequently, a vitamin D deficiency may result in a pro-inflammatory phenotype, which could increase the severity of the disease. To better understand how vitamin D might influence these and other important pathways during infection, more research is required.

AUTISM

Can autism in some form be brought on by inadequate vitamin D during pregnancy and infancy?

Some researchers believe the response is YES.

The common neurodevelopmental disorder known as autism spectrum disorder (ASD) is brought on by a complex interplay between genetic and environmental risk factors. Given that vitamin D3 (cholecalciferol) is crucial for brain development, it appears to be one of the environmental factors that significantly contributes to the etiology of ASD. Lower vitamin D3 levels have been linked to larger brains, altered brain shapes, and enlarged ventricles, which have been seen in ASD patients. In the liver, vitamin D3 is changed into 25-hydroxyvitamin D3. Increased levels of this steroid in the serum may lower the risk of autism. It's important to note that children with ASD are more likely to suffer from vitamin D deficiency, possibly as a result of environmental factors. Additionally, a lack of vitamin D3 has been linked to ASD symptoms.

Autism cannot be cured, but vitamin D may help lessen the severity of the symptoms. It might aid in restoring some neural and brain functions to normal. Additionally, it can reduce inflammation.

EPILEPSY

Vitamin D3 may lessen seizures in animal models and open-label clinical trials, according to preclinical and early clinical research. Vitamin D3 is a fascinating candidate in the search for complementary epilepsy treatments. Christiansen first proposed that vitamin D supplementation might raise calcium and magnesium levels while lowering hyperexcitability in epilepsy patients as early as 1974.

DIABETES

Vitamin D reduced the risk of diabetes by 15%, with an absolute risk reduction of 3.3% over three years. They discovered that, in people with prediabetes, vitamin D was helpful in lowering the risk for diabetes and increasing the likelihood of regression to normal glucose regulation, with no opposing safety signals.

The generalizability of these results is constrained, though. First, trials with vitamin D that were directed at children, pregnant or lactating women, patients who were in hospitals, and patients with end-stage renal disease or HIV at enrollment were not included in the initial search.

These results do not currently apply to the general healthy population or people at average risk for type 2, type 1, or other types of diabetes because the study population included people at high risk of type 2 diabetes.

OBESITY

When compared to their non-obese counterparts, obese men's vitamin D intake has been found to be lower, but not for women. Obesity has also been linked to low calcium and vitamin D intake in both men and women, but this correlation does not necessarily imply causation.

ASTHMA

Asthma and vitamin D are becoming more and more associated. Lower levels of inflammatory markers and reduced airway hyperresponsiveness are linked to higher vitamin D levels. Poor asthma control and increased severity may be linked to low vitamin D levels. Asthma patients had low vitamin D levels. Following vitamin D supplementation, there was a highly significant improvement in asthma control and severity. When taken within six months of the follow-up period, especially in children, vitamin D supplements can reduce asthma flare-ups. Numerous studies have shown that people with low vitamin D levels are more likely to experience asthma flare-ups.

According to research, children who had non-smoking parents had significantly higher vitamin D levels than kids who had both smoking parents. Children who had only one parent who smoked either maternally or paternally had intermediate vitamin D levels.

ECZEMA

The most prevalent skin condition in the entire world is eczema (atopic dermatitis). Around 20% of children and 5% of adults are affected, and symptoms can range from minor annoyances to serious setbacks that affect your confidence.

Due to its ability to support your skin barrier and immune system, vitamin D supplements and direct sun exposure are linked to reduced eczema symptoms.

When scientists discovered that people who lived in areas with less sunlight had higher rates of both eczema and vitamin D deficiency, they made the connection between vitamin D and eczema.

According to one study, children's symptoms were better when they spent more time in the sun than when they remained in a colder, darker environment. More recently, a meta-analysis (a thorough review of a collection of studies on vitamin D and eczema) came to the conclusion that vitamin D significantly reduced the severity of eczema symptoms in all of the studies it included.

The severity of eczema was found to be lessened by taking vitamin D for two months in several studies on adults. Even better outcomes may be achieved, particularly in cases of severe symptoms, by combining vitamin D with other nutrients that support the skin, such as vitamin E, or by taking it concurrently with eczema medications.

It might strengthen the area of your immune system in charge of maintaining the integrity of your skin barrier. The first line of defense against the outside world is this barrier. Although vitamin D receptors assist in controlling particular proteins that fortify your skin barrier, people with eczema have abnormal skin barrier function.

Studies have shown a correlation between higher eczema rates and lower vitamin D levels, particularly in children. When compared to children without skin conditions, children with moderate to severe eczema are more likely to have lower vitamin D levels, particularly if they have lighter skin tones.

ACNE

Here is what is currently known about the relationship between vitamin D and acne, though more research is being done in this area. According to a 2015 study, those with cystic acne who had low vitamin D levels were more likely to experience more severe signs and symptoms. Another study discovered that taking oral vitamin D supplements significantly reduced the severity of acne-related symptoms in participants. In other words, acne may be more likely to occur in people who are vitamin D deficient.

HEALING OF WOUNDS

By interacting with the vitamin D receptor (VDR) through calcitriol, vitamin D aids in wound healing. By promoting the production of mitogenic growth factors and receptors like platelet-derived growth factor (PDGF), epidermal growth factor receptors (EGFR), and keratinocyte growth factor receptor (KGFR), it controls the transcription downstream in various target cells. Calcium and vitamin D are two essential regulators of these skin-related processes. Calcium and vitamin D help to create the permeability barrier, which prevents fluid loss and boosts the innate immune response, which guards against infection.

Numerous patients with chronic wounds are found to be vitamin D deficient, and dressings containing calcium and vitamin D are effective. This suggests that further research into the mechanisms by which calcium and vitamin D signaling promote wound healing will have a significant clinical impact on this population. Supplementation has proven effective in the oral mucosa's wound-healing processes.

ANEMIA

Recent developments in our knowledge of the relationship between vitamin D and anemia lead us to believe that maintaining adequate vitamin D status may be crucial for preventing anemia, particularly in conditions marked by inflammation. Early clinical trials have been encouraging, but more studies are required to determine whether vitamin D will be an effective treatment for anemia in the future.

Anemia, especially anemia of inflammation, may benefit from vitamin D's down-regulatory effects on inflammatory cytokines and hepcidin.

BONE HEALTH

If your bones hurt when you press on them, you probably don't get enough vitamin D.

Strong muscles and bones require vitamin D. Our bodies cannot effectively absorb calcium, which is necessary for strong bones, without vitamin D.

Rickets, a condition that results in weak bones, bowed legs, and other skeletal deformities like stooped posture in children, is brought on by vitamin D deficiency.

Recent research has suggested that vitamin D may play a role in preventing fractures by mediating effects on inflammation and muscle function (a defect in muscle function is one of the classic signs of rickets). Studies have shown that vitamin D supplementation can increase muscle strength, which in turn helps to reduce the likelihood of falls, one of the leading causes of fractures. Pro-inflammatory cytokines have been linked to increased bone metabolism, and osteoporosis is frequently thought to be an inflammatory condition. Thus, the impact of these cytokines on bone health and subsequent fracture risk may be modulated by the immunoregulatory mechanisms of vitamin D. Therefore, a variety of mechanisms by which vitamin D may affect fracture risk.

SLEEP

The quantity and quality of your sleep will be impacted if you don't get enough vitamin D.

In the control of sleep, vitamin D plays both a direct and an indirect role. Although vitamin D deficiency has been linked to sleep disorders, there is still little evidence to conclusively support the prevention or treatment of sleep disturbances with vitamin D supplements; more intervention studies are actually required to better understand these concepts.

Our entire body, including the central nervous system, contains vitamin D receptors. These receptors manage your sleep cycle and aid in getting a good night's rest so you can wake up feeling rested. However, these receptors are unable to perform as intended because of the amount deficit. Another factor is that low vitamin D levels cause higher cortisol levels, or the stress hormone, which makes it difficult to fall asleep.

Severe sleep disorders like insomnia and sleep apnea could dcvclop from these ongoing sleep problems.

MIGRAINE AND HEADACHE

Some supplements may be beneficial for migraine sufferers' health. A migraine attack may be brought on by vitamin deficiency, particularly magnesium and vitamin D deficiency. This is most likely a result of its function in battling brain inflammation. Additionally, vitamin D may increase the absorption of magnesium and decrease the synthesis of substances that rise during migraine attacks.

Supplementing with vitamin D may be helpful in treating and preventing migraines, especially in those who are vitamin D deficient. A lack of vitamin D has been linked to migraines, and it may prevent headaches in a number of different ways.

Getting enough vitamin D may help shield you from migraines.

DEPRESSION

According to the National Health and Nutrition Examination Survey, those who don't get enough vitamin D are much more likely to experience depression than those who do. According to a Dutch study, people with depression had 14% lower levels of vitamin D (1,25-hydroxyvitamin D, a form of vitamin D) in their blood than people without the diagnosis.

FATIGUE

You should not ignore a sign that you are constantly tired. There is a common vitamin D deficiency that has been linked in uncontrolled studies to fatigue.

In otherwise healthy individuals with vitamin D deficiency, treatment with vitamin D significantly reduced fatigue.

In primary care settings in both developed and developing nations, fatigue is a common complaint. It may result in lowered quality of life and lost time at the office. In order to presumptively treat the symptom, doctors are likely to prescribe vitamins, especially vitamin D, iron, and nutritional supplements.

LIFESPAN

Recent developments in vitamin D research suggest that, in addition to the musculoskeletal system, this secosteroid hormone also benefits other body systems. The active hormonal form of vitamin D, 1,25-dihydroxyvitamin D [1,25(OH)2D], as well as 25 dihydroxyvitamin D [25(OH)2D], are both crucial for maintaining healthy physiology in humans, including reducing inflammation and excessive intracellular oxidative stresses.

One of the most important regulators of systemic inflammation, oxidative stress, mitochondrial respiratory function, and consequently human aging is vitamin D. In turn, 1,25(OH)2D's molecular and cellular actions lessen oxidative stress, cell and tissue damage, and aging. Conversely, hypovitaminosis D worsens oxidative stress and systemic inflammation while impairing mitochondrial functions.

The interaction of 1,25(OH)2D with its intracellular receptors modifies the transcription of genes that are dependent on vitamin D and activates elements that are responsive to it, which sets off a variety of second messenger systems. Therefore, it should come as no surprise that hypovitaminosis D raises the prevalence and severity of a number of age-related common diseases, including metabolic conditions associated with oxidative stress. These include autoimmune diseases, certain cancers, obesity, insulin resistance, type 2 diabetes, hypertension, pregnancy complications, memory issues, osteoporosis, and systemic inflammatory diseases.

Adequate vitamin D reduces oxidative stress, enhances mitochondrial and endocrine functions, and lowers the risk of diseases like autoimmunity, infections, metabolic disturbances, and DNA repair impairment. All of these factors contribute to a healthy, graceful aging process. Protein oxidation, lipid peroxidation, and DNA damage caused by oxidative stress are all prevented by vitamin D's strong antioxidant properties, which promote balanced mitochondrial activities.

PREGNANCY

Every person needs vitamin D because it assists in the appropriate absorption of calcium and phosphate. It is especially crucial during pregnancy because it promotes the growth of your unborn child's bones, teeth, kidneys, heart, and nervous system.

Every day, pregnant women should supplement with 10 micrograms (or 400 IU) of vitamin D. Your baby will receive enough vitamin D from this for the first few months of life.

You run the risk of giving birth to a child with soft bones if you do not take a vitamin D supplement during pregnancy. Rickets, a condition that affects a child's ability to develop bones, may result from this.

SKIN

Did you know that vitamin D is crucial for the health of your skin in addition to your bones and immune system? Dryness, redness, psoriasis, and eczema are a few of the skin issues that are linked to vitamin D deficiency. Fortunately, increasing your vitamin D levels can have a significant impact on your skin's appearance and health as well as the condition of your hair.

Vitamin D is essential for healthy skin because it:

- Maintains a barrier against sun damage
- controls the cellular replication cycle, preventing early aging

- Antioxidant defenses are boosted to combat dangerous free radicals.
- encourages the production of collagen, which helps skin cells take shape and be strong.

Because it aids in controlling blood calcium levels, vitamin D is crucial for the health of the skin. Calcium is essential for keeping skin hydrated and infection-free. Hyaluronic acid, a naturally occurring compound that aids in the retention of water in the skin and gives it a more hydrated and youthful appearance, is also stimulated by vitamin D in skin cells.

Since vitamin D is naturally produced in the body when we are exposed to the sun's ultraviolet rays, sun exposure is a good way to obtain it. In fact, research has shown that exposure to the sun improves skin tone and elasticity while preventing premature skin aging.

SAFETY OF VITAMIN D

How much is excessive?

When taken in moderation, vitamin D is regarded as safe. However, supplementing with excessive amounts of vitamin D can be harmful.

Children older than 9, adults, pregnant women, and nursing mothers who take more than 4,000 IU of vitamin D daily may experience nausea and vomiting, according to the National Health Institute. loss of weight and poor appetite, Weakness, diarrhea, confusion, and disorientation, cardiac rhythm issues, kidney damage, and kidney stones.

BEST VITAMIN D LEVEL

The following vitamin D dosages should be consumed each day, according to the National Institutes of Health (NIH)Trusted Source:

AGE	AMOUNT (MALE OR FEMALE)
0–12 months	10 micrograms (400 IU)
1–70 years	15 micrograms (600 IU)
71 years and above	20 micrograms (800 IU)

The precise quantity of vitamin D you will require, either from your diet or from supplements, depends on a variety of variables:

- Age
- Skin tone, which reflects the amount of melanin in the skin
- The latitude where you live

- Season
- Sun exposure
- Your clothing choices
- Whether or not you are obese

CHAPTER TWO

VITAMIN C

Vitamin C, also known as ascorbic acid is a water-soluble vitamin. It can be delivered to the body's tissues by dissolving in water, but because it cannot be effectively stored, it must be consumed daily through food or supplements. Nutritionists knew something in citrus fruits could prevent scurvy, a condition that may have killed up to two million sailors between 1500 and 1800, even before its discovery in 1932.

Citrus fruits, tomatoes, red and green peppers, liver (27 mg), steak (25 mg), berries, broccoli, and apple juice are all sources of vitamin C.

Vitamin C is a potent antioxidant that can disarm dangerous free radicals and aid in the healing of wounds and infections. It is required for the production of collagen, a fibrous protein found in connective tissue and woven throughout the nervous, immune, bone, cartilage, blood, and other systems in the body.

It also supports the production of various hormones and chemical messengers that are used in the brain and nerves.

CANCER

Because of its general characteristics or because of its function as an antioxidant, vitamin C is linked to the treatment of cancer. Some medical professionals think cancer cells are killed by vitamin C therapy. It might also function as an antioxidant, defending against the harm caused by free radicals, according to researchers at the National Institutes of Health.

In the same way that chemotherapy produces hydrogen peroxide, intravenous vitamin C also kills cancer cells by causing oxidative damage to them. This is how intravenous vitamin C works on cancer cells.

For this, vitamin C must be administered intravenously; otherwise, the body will simply regulate the amount of vitamin C consumed orally and eliminate any excess through urination.

It can be used in conjunction with conventional chemo and radiation but only in extremely high intravenous doses. For those who don't respond to other treatments, it's a great option. However, there is no guarantee that it will apply to everyone.

DENTAL HEALTH

By strengthening the oral mucous membranes and assisting in the fight against specific types of bacteria that can lead to tooth decay, vitamin C promotes healthy teeth and gums. Additionally, vitamin C may help guard against gum disease by limiting the development of bacteria that cause plaque, thereby reducing gum inflammation and bleeding.

According to some studies, vitamin C may help people with chronic dry mouth caused by drugs or other conditions like Sjogren's syndrome. This is due to the fact that vitamin C encourages salivation, which keeps your mouth moist and inhibits the growth of harmful bacteria on your tongue or in your mouth.

The soft tissues in your mouth and your gums are fortified by vitamin C. It can protect you from gingivitis, the early stages of gum disease, and stop your teeth from becoming loose.

INFECTION

In the early literature, vitamin C inadequacy was linked with pneumonia. After its recognition, an amount of studies enquired the effects of vitamin C on various infections. A sum of 148 animal studies revealed that vitamin C may lessen or inhibit infections caused by bacteria, viruses, and protozoa. The most thoroughly studied human infection is the common cold. Vitamin C administration does not decrease the average incidence of colds in the general population, yet it halves the number of colds in physically active people. Continuously administered vitamin C has shortened the span of colds, pointing to a biological effect.

PAIN

The vitamin C deficiency disease scurvy is characterized by musculoskeletal pain and recent epidemiological evidence has indicated an association between suboptimal vitamin C status and spinal pain.

In addition, accumulated evidence shows that vitamin C administration can exhibit analgesic properties in a considerable amount of clinical conditions.
The prevalence of hypovitaminosis C and vitamin C inadequacy is high in numerous patient groups, such as surgical/trauma, infectious diseases, and cancer patients.

A number of current clinical studies have revealed that vitamin C administration to patients with chronic regional pain syndrome alleviates their symptoms. Acute herpetic and post-herpetic neuralgia is also reduced with high dose vitamin C administration

Additionally, a high dose of vitamin C reduces cancer-related pain, improving patient quality of life. The analgesic effects of vitamin C have been attributed to a variety of mechanisms.

In general, vitamin C appears to be a secure and efficient adjunctive therapy for the treatment of acute and chronic pain in particular patient populations.

DIABETES

According to the research, those with type 2 diabetes who took a vitamin C supplement for four months had lower post-meal blood sugar levels than those who took a placebo.

OBESITY

One of the biggest health risks in the world today is obesity. Additionally, the excessive accumulation of body fat that characterizes this condition may cause a number of clinical manifestations that are related to it, including cardiovascular problems, type 2 diabetes, inflammation, and some forms of cancer. These comorbidities' emergence has frequently been linked to unbalanced oxidative stress. Antioxidant-based therapies could therefore be thought of as intriguing means of preventing the complications associated with obesity-related fat accumulation.

Ascorbic acid, a form of vitamin C, has been found to have a negative correlation with the development of a number of diseases including hypertension, gallbladder disease, stroke, cancer, atherosclerosis, as well as obesity in both humans and animals. It has been proposed that ascorbic acid may have the following positive effects on mechanisms relating to obesity:

- Modulate adipocyte lipolysis
- Control the release of glucocorticoids from adrenal glands
- Slow down glucose metabolism and leptin secretion on isolated adipocytes.
- Improve hyperglycemia and reduce glycosylation in obese-diabetic models
- Lessen the inflammatory response.

All of these qualities might be connected to this vitamin's exceptional antioxidant properties.

DEPRESSION

Citalopram's effectiveness in treating patients with MDD (major depressive disorder) was not increased by adding vitamin C to it. When used in combination with citalopram, vitamin C is just as effective as a placebo in treating suicidal behavior in adult patients. During this trial, no significant adverse effects of this combination were found.

INFERTILITY

You might be trying to increase your fertility if you're trying to get pregnant. Vitamin C is one nutrient that you might want to think about.

Strong antioxidant vitamin C is essential for several bodily functions, including collagen synthesis, wound healing, and immune system operation. As an antioxidant, it can aid in defending the egg against oxidative stress damage.

The quality of cervical mucus may be enhanced by vitamin C, making it simpler for sperm to reach the egg.

Male fertility may also benefit from vitamin C. Oxidative stress can harm sperm in particular, which can lower their quality and make it more difficult for them to fertilize an egg.

Antioxidant qualities of vitamin C can aid in shielding sperm from this harm and enhancing their general quality.

BONE

Vitamin C, which has historically been linked to scurvy, is a crucial nutrient for preserving bone health. It is necessary for the synthesis of collagen in the bone matrix. Additionally, it scavenges free radicals bad for bone health.

CATARACTS

The most common reason for blindness worldwide is cataracts or clouding of the lens. Age and diabetes are significant risk factors, and the prevalence of cataracts will rise as more people age and develop diabetes.

Although cataract surgery is a successful method for restoring vision, there must also be other options if the looming cataract epidemic is to be stopped. Antioxidants have been promoted as treatments to postpone and/or prevent cataracts because it is well-established that oxidative damage plays a significant part in the etiology of cataracts.

As cataract treatments, many antioxidant interventions, including vitamin C, have yielded contradictory results. In order to address some of the discrepancies found in previous animal and human studies, progress has been made in our understanding of lens physiology and the mechanisms involved in the uptake and delivery of antioxidants to the lens.

The possibility of vitamin C-based supplements postponing the development of cataracts after vitrectomy, which happens in up to 80% of patients within two years, is intriguing. These focused strategies are necessary to lessen the impact of cataracts on hospitals and raise the standard of living for our elderly and diabetic population.

ALLERGIES

Ascorbic acid, also known as vitamin C, may help with some allergies, according to some evidence. Antioxidant and natural antihistamine properties of vitamin C. According to studies, it might lessen the swelling, inflammation, and other symptoms that appear at the site of an allergic reaction.

Your immune system's response to an allergen, also known as an invader, causes allergy symptoms. Pollen, pet dander, and the proteins in some foods are examples of common allergens.

Most cells, which are immune system cells that release histamine when activated, work to help block the invader.

The following allergic symptoms could be aggravated by histamine:

- Runny nose
- Sneezing
- Red and watery eyes
- Itching
- Rash
- Asthma
- Vomiting or diarrhea
- Swelling
- Anaphylaxis; a rare but deadly swelling in the airway

Antihistamine medications can block histamine and its effects for mild seasonal or environmental allergies, but they can also have their own undesirable side effects.

In contrast to antihistamine drugs, vitamin C works by lowering the amount of histamine your body produces rather than by blocking histamine receptors.

According to research, taking 2 grams of vitamin C may cause a person's histamine levels to drop by about 38%.

A higher dose of vitamin C administered intravenously might be more efficient. According to a small study involving 89 individuals with allergies or infectious diseases, those who received a 7.5-gram intravenous (IV) vitamin C infusion had roughly 50% less histamine in their blood.

According to the study, those with allergies benefited more from a decrease in histamine than those with infectious diseases.

Another observational study examined the results of giving people with allergic symptoms of the skin or respiratory system an intravenous (IV) infusion of vitamin C. It was discovered that in 97% of allergy sufferers, a 7.5-gram dose administered intravenously was linked to a decrease in allergy symptoms like runny nose, sneezing, itching, restlessness, and sleep issues. Out of 71 people, only 1 reported any negative effects.

A vitamin C nasal spray was also put to the test in a high-quality study on 60 people who had allergy symptoms like runny nose and sneezing. According to the study, symptoms were 74% better.

BITES

The proteolytic activity of the venom from Echis carinatus was significantly and dose-dependently inhibited by ascorbic acid. Isothermal titration calorimetry interaction studies of ascorbic acid with purified ecarin revealed favorable binding energy and energetics.

Ascorbic acid's molecular docking with ecarin revealed significant interactions with residues in the protein's active site pocket. The ligand was found to act as a chelating inhibitor. As a result, the ascorbic acid backbone structural scaffold has the potential to be used as a building block in the development of drug-like molecules for the treatment of viper bites.

Banana peel interiors are rich in vitamin C, an antihistamine that is excellent for treating insect bites and has antibacterial properties.

SKIN

Antioxidants of vitamin C may aid in protecting against the possible harm that UV light can do. This does not imply that a vitamin C skin serum can take the place of sunscreen. Since it doesn't block UVA or UVB rays, it can't be used in place of SPF.

However, if UV light does penetrate your skin, some research indicates that vitamin C may be able to lessen the damage.

Hyperpigmented patches of your skin, also known as hyperpigmentation, may become lighter with the use of vitamin C-based skin care products. In one study, spots were significantly reduced after 16 weeks of vitamin C application to the skin.

In many anti-aging products, vitamin C is a potent ingredient. According to some studies, using it consistently for at least 12 weeks can help reduce the visibility of wrinkles. Additionally, a nutritious diet rich in this nutrient may be beneficial. According to research, people who consume more vitamin C are less likely to wrinkle. Not just citrus fruits can be used for it. It is also found in copious supply in spinach, red peppers, and broccoli.

LIFESPAN

It has been discovered that vitamin C lowers the risk of early death from cancer, cardiovascular disease, and compromised immune systems. People with the highest blood levels of vitamin C showed a 25% lower risk of dying from any cause in a recent study. According to research, vitamin C helps people live longer and can fend off many aging-related diseases, including cancer. A significant new study found that people with higher blood levels of vitamin C had significantly lower risks of dying from cancer and heart disease, as well as up to 25% lower risks of dying from any cause. The quality of life could be significantly enhanced by vitamin C.

SAFETY OF VITAMIN C

Supplemental vitamin C has a diuretic effect, assisting the body in eliminating extra water. When taking them, be sure to drink plenty of water. The majority of commercial vitamin C is produced from corn. People who are allergic to corn should look for alternatives, like sago palm.

The amount of iron absorbed from food is increased by vitamin C. Vitamin C supplements shouldn't be taken by people with hemochromatosis, an inherited condition in which the body accumulates too much iron.

Because your body eliminates any excess vitamin C, it is generally thought to be safe. However, at high doses (more than 2,000 mg per day), it can result in gas, bloating, or stomach discomfort. Reduce the vitamin C dosage if you experience these side effects.

Before taking vitamin C, people with kidney issues should speak to their doctor.

Because nicotine reduces vitamin C's bioavailability in the body, people who smoke or use nicotine patches may require more vitamin C.

Because their intake of vitamin C drops after giving birth, babies born to mothers who consume 6,000 mg or more of vitamin C are at risk for rebound scurvy. Consult your doctor before taking more than 1,000 mg of vitamin C if you are pregnant.

High doses of vitamin C have the potential to cause serious side effects in people with sickle cell anemia and G6PD, a metabolic disorder.

Patients with hemochromatosis and thalassemia may experience adverse effects from increased iron absorption, which may result from vitamin C supplementation.

In diabetics, vitamin C may cause blood sugar levels to rise. Vitamin C intakes above 300 mg per day were linked to an increased risk of death from heart disease in older women with diabetes.

Vitamin C consumption immediately before or after angioplasty may hinder healing.

Before taking vitamin C, consult your oncologist if you are undergoing cancer treatment. Some chemotherapy drugs and vitamin C might interact.

BEST VITAMIN C LEVEL

For adults aged 19 and older, the recommended daily allowance is 90 mg for men and 75 mg for women.

The dosage rises to 85 mg and 120 mg daily for pregnancy and lactation, respectively. An additional 35 mg of vitamin C above the RDA is advised for smokers because smoking can reduce the body's vitamin C levels.

The daily intake amount that is least likely to have a negative impact on health is known as the Tolerable Upper Intake Level. The UL for vitamin C is 2000 mg per day; exceeding this amount may encourage diarrhea and gastrointestinal distress. Only under specific conditions, such as in controlled clinical trials or when supervised by a physician, are doses greater than the UL occasionally used.

The ability of the intestines to absorb vitamin C is constrained. According to studies, taking more than 1000 mg of vitamin C reduces absorption by less than 50%. Megadoses of vitamin C are not toxic in generally healthy adults because absorption decreases once the body's tissues are saturated with the vitamin and any extra is excreted in the urine. With the quantity taken in exceeding 3000 mg per day, side-effects are however possible. These include reports of diarrhea, an increased risk of kidney stones developing in people with kidney disease or a history of stones, elevated uric acid levels (a risk factor for gout), and raised iron absorption and overload in people with hemochromatosis, a hereditary condition that arises in excessive iron in the blood.

Getting the RDA or slightly more vitamin C may offer protection against certain disease states because vitamin C is involved in a number of metabolic processes in the body. Larger doses have not been found to have any health benefits in individuals who are generally in good health and have adequate nutrition. According to cell studies, vitamin C can switch from being an antioxidant to a tissue-damaging pro-oxidant at very high concentrations. It can increase the risk of kidney stones and digestive problems in humans, but its effects at doses far above the RDA are unknown.

CHAPTER THREE

IODINE

The thyroid uses an element called iodine. Iodine must be consumed because it cannot be produced by humans. Salt and some foods both contain it as an ingredient.

Fungi, bacteria, and other microorganisms like amoebas can all be killed by iodine. One of the most prevalent and curable health issues in the entire world is iodine deficiency. The majority of iodine can be found in oceans, where it is primarily concentrated by sea life, especially seaweed.

Iodine is a trace element that is required in the proper concentration but not in large amounts. It can be found as a dietary supplement and is naturally added to some salts and some foods. Thyroxine (T4) and triiodothyronine (T3) both require iodine as a necessary component. The thyroid is the body's biggest iodine consumer. Thyroid hormones are crucial regulators of metabolic activity and control a variety of significant biochemical processes, such as protein synthesis and enzymatic activity. They are also necessary for a fetus's and an infant's proper skeletal and nervous system development.

CANCER

All of the iodine in your body is absorbed almost entirely by your thyroid gland. Because of this, thyroid cancer can be treated with radioactive iodine (RAI, also known as I-131). With little impact on the rest of your body, the RAI primarily accumulates in thyroid cells, where the radiation can kill the thyroid gland and any additional thyroid cells (including cancer cells) that take up iodine.

When papillary or follicular thyroid cancer (differentiated thyroid cancer) has spread to the neck or other body parts, radioactive iodine therapy, which is now standard practice in such cases, helps patients live longer. The advantages of RAI therapy, however, are less obvious for those who have small thyroid cancers that can frequently be completely removed through surgery and do not appear to have spread. With your doctor, go over the risks and advantages of RAI therapy. Anaplastic (undifferentiated) and medullary thyroid cancer cannot be treated with radioactive iodine therapy because they do not absorb iodine.

BREAST HEALTH

Iodine's role in breast health, particularly the positive effects it has shown in relation to breast cancer risk, fibrocystic breast disease, premenstrual breast tenderness, and mammary dysplasia, may be one of the most exciting and interesting areas of iodine research. Iodine has been shown to have antioxidant properties in the breasts, which means it helps prevent cellular damage. This may help to partially explain why diets high in iodine are linked to a lower risk of breast cancer. Iodine is also known to prevent the growth of abnormal cells and to encourage the development of normal breast tissue.

Iodine deficiency is linked to an increased risk of fibrocystic breast disease, a condition characterized by lumpiness in one or both breasts, in addition to breast cancer risk. Up to 50% of women of reproductive age are affected by fibrocystic breast disease, but fortunately, iodine supplementation has been shown to be effective in treating the disease. If you experience lumpiness or discomfort in one or both of your breasts, it is important to have it looked into. If fibrocystic breast disease is found to be the cause, working with a naturopath or other healthcare professional who can look into the possibility of iodine deficiency as a contributing factor may be beneficial.

HEART VALVE HEALTH

A higher iodine intake may improve cardiovascular function because iodine deficiency can have harmful effects on the cardiovascular system. Public health organizations have aggressively promoted sodium restriction as a way to lower blood pressure and the risk of cardiovascular disease in recent years. In many developed countries, these incentives have caused an overall decline in the consumption of iodine. For instance, 1 in 40 participants in a national health survey of the United States in the early 1970s had urinary iodine levels that were suggestive of moderate or greater iodine deficiency; 20 years later, 1 in 9 participants had moderate to severe iodine deficiency.

The prevalence of hypothyroidism and hyperthyroidism has been linked to regional iodine intake, with autoimmune hypothyroidism being the more prevalent of the two in areas with moderate to high iodine intake. It has been demonstrated that both of these thyroid abnormalities are detrimental to cardiovascular health.

Selenium, a crucial antioxidant in the thyroid that is also involved in the metabolism of thyroid hormones containing iodine, may interact with these thyroid irregularities to cause cardiovascular disease. Cardiovascular disease and hypertension have long been treated with iodine and iodine-rich foods.

PREGNANCY

Reduced fertility is linked to iodine deficiency. Recent studies have shown that couples with unexplained infertility (UI) have higher conception rates when using contrast media with high iodine concentrations. We speculate that this improvement may be due to the excess iodine and mechanisms other than its effects on the thyroid.

During pregnancy, iodine requirements are increased by about 50%. Iodine deficiency during pregnancy can affect the fetus's ability to develop neurologically and result in hypothyroidism in both the mother and the fetus. The effects are dependent on the severity and timing of the hypothyroidism; cretinism is the most severe symptom. Iodine supplementation before or during early pregnancy in iodine-deficient areas has been shown to eliminate new cases of cretinism, increase birth weight, lower rates of perinatal and infant mortality, and generally increase developmental scores in young children by 10–20%.

Although mild-to-moderate maternal iodine deficiency can lead to thyroid dysfunction, it is unclear whether this affects the children's cognitive and/or neurological development. The most affordable method of delivering iodine and enhancing maternal and infant health in nearly all areas with iodine deficiency is salt iodization.

IMMUNITY

Iodine (I) is a trace element that is necessary for both humans and animals, and a lack of it can impair the immune system and basal metabolism. Iodine deficiency causes physical illnesses and weakened immune systems in large numbers of people worldwide.

Iodine deficiency is one of the most significant nutritional factors that have a significant impact on the health status of the population, particularly children at all stages of development, according to the United Nations Children's Fund (UNICEF) and World Health Organization (WHO). Iodine is used in cell-mediated immunity by the enzyme leukocyte myeloperoxidase to produce iodine-free radicals.

Myeloperoxidase, which is also present in thyroid cells, oxidizes tyrosine to a tyrosyl radical using hydrogen peroxide, and its inactivity predisposes to immune deficiency. Its concentration is highest in granulocytes and lowest in lymphocytes.

The immune suppression impairs cytokine production and reduces the acute-phase response to infections, which has an adverse impact on the course of inflammatory diseases. It was demonstrated in 2013 that iodine treatment led to fewer lung lesions and less pulmonary expression of RSV antigen in newborn lambs who had received an RSV vaccination. Additionally, it was shown that iodine supplementation lessened the severity of RSV infection in 3-week-old lambs.

Studies have revealed the special characteristics of iodine germicide. Furthermore, numerous studies have shown that Tasco-Forage, a (iodine-rich) extract from the brown seaweed Ascophyllum nodosum, boosts the immune system and antioxidant activity in grazing animals.

Iodine's crucial role in boosting the immune system, combating the virus, and subsequent anti-inflammatory properties make it potentially effective in the fight against COVID-19.

Consequently, it offers a practical, cost-effective, and reasonable solution for the control and treatment of COVID-19 prior to the peak of vaccine production.

NEURODEVELOPMENT

The synthesis of thyroid hormones needs iodine. The development of the brain takes place during fetal and early postnatal life, and these hormones are necessary for that process.

The thyroid gland produces the hormone thyroxin, which is made from the element iodine. Iodine deficiency is currently the single biggest contributor to mental retardation because both iodine and thyroxine are necessary for brain development. It is also the one cause that is most easily avoidable. Iodine deficiency has been linked to problems with child survival and development, according to numerous studies.

IODINE SAFETY

Iodine controls metabolism, the process by which food energy is transformed into energy that supports cellular growth and function. Therefore, normal growth and development can be hampered by an iodine deficiency.

This can lead to miscarriage, stillbirth, stunted growth, and cognitive impairments (difficulties with reading, writing, talking, problem-solving, and social skills), which are particularly dangerous in pregnant women and infants. Iodine deficiency in children has also been linked to a lower IQ, according to research. Iodine inadequacy in adults of less than 10 to 20 mcg per day can cause hypothyroidism, which affects normal metabolic processes like controlling body weight, heart rate, and body temperature. Goiters, a lump or swelling in the neck, frequently accompany hypothyroidism. Additional indications of hypothyroidism include:

- Weakness Fatigue
- Cold sensitivity
- Constipation
- Dry hair and skin
- gaining weight

Those who do not use iodized salt or iodine supplements, pregnant women, vegans who do not consume any animal products, and residents of areas with low soil iodine levels (such as mountainous areas) are all at risk for iodine deficiency.

Most healthy individuals can tolerate high iodine intakes without any issues. This has been noticed in nations that regularly consume iodine-rich seaweed, like Japan and Korea. However, some individuals with autoimmune thyroid disease or those who have a history of chronic iodine deficiency may be sensitive to extra iodine, leading to iodine deficiency conditions like hypothyroidism and goiter. The condition known as hyperthyroidism, which has symptoms including a fast or irregular heartbeat, hand tremors, irritability, fatigue, and perspiration, can also be brought on by too much iodine in the body. In some sensitive people, even a small excess of dietary iodine over the RDA can result in iodine-induced hyperthyroidism.

High seaweed consumption has been linked to an increased risk of some thyroid cancers, particularly in postmenopausal women, according to some epidemiologic studies, but the precise mechanism is still unknown.

The use of high-dose supplements or excessive consumption of some seaweeds and salts that contain iodine can result in excessive iodine intake. Although it is uncommon, severe iodine poisoning can cause a coma as well as symptoms like fever, stomach pain, nausea, vomiting, and a burning sensation in the mouth, throat, and stomach. Iodine toxicity, iodine-induced hypothyroidism, and hyperthyroidism are particularly dangerous for children, infants, the elderly, and people who already have thyroid disease.

BEST IODINE LEVEL

Your stage of life will determine how much iodine you require each day.

LIFE STAGE	RECOMMENDED DAILY INTAKE
Babies 0 –6 months	110 micrograms
Babies 7–12 months	130 micrograms
Children aged 1–8	90 micrograms
Children aged 9–13	120 micrograms
Teenagers aged 14–18	150 micrograms
Adults	150 micrograms
Pregnant women	220 micrograms
Breastfeeding women	290 micrograms

The daily dose that is most likely to prevent adverse side effects in the general population is known as a Tolerable Upper Intake Level (UL).
The recommended daily intake of iodine for adults, pregnant women, and nursing mothers is 1,100 mcg.

CONCLUSION

As you can see, iodine, vitamin C, and vitamin D are crucial nutrients required for survival and good health. Remember to buy foods that contain these ingredients the next time you go grocery shopping.

You should be aware that you might not be getting enough of these nutrients from your diet to meet your body's needs. You can fix this by purchasing supplements of these nutrients to ensure you are getting the right amount but don't overdo it.

Most importantly, try exposing yourself to the summer sun during midday. It has been demonstrated that 20 minutes of summertime midday sun can produce up to 20,000 IU of vitamin D.